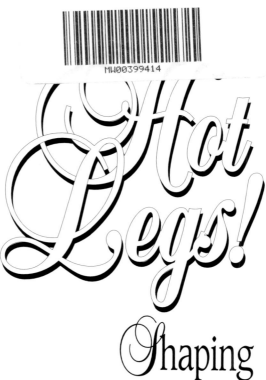

Hot Legs!

Shaping
A Tight
& Trim
Lower
Body

Published by MuscleMag International
6465 Airport Road
Mississauga, ON
Canada L4V 1E4

Designed by Jackie Kydyk
Edited by Mandy Morgan

Canadian Cataloguing in Publication Data

Kennedy, Robert, 1938-
    Hot legs! : shaping a tight & trim lower body

ISBN 1-55210-009-X

    1. Exercise for women. 2. Leg.
I. Hines Dwayne, 1961- II. Title.

GV546.6.W64K45 1998   613.7'045   C97-901234-1

10 9 8 7 6 5 4 3 2

Distributed in Canada by
CANBOOK Distribution Services
1220 Nicholson Road
Newmarket, ON
L3Y 7V1
1-800-399-6858

Distributed in the United States by
BookWorld Services
1933 Whitfield Park Loop
Sarasota, FL 34243
1-800-444-2524

Printed in Canada

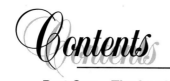Contents

Part One THE LEG WORKOUT

Legs – like them or not, you have a pair. Your legs are essential for getting you where you want to go. And your legs are more than just a pair of "wheels" – they also play a large role in communicating the state of your physique. Your lower body makes up more than half of your body structure, and your leg muscles are the largest muscle group of your entire physique. If you want to change the shape of your body, you have to pay particular attention to your legs.

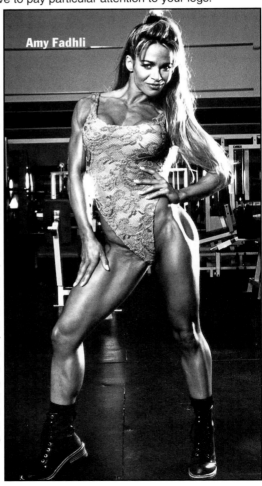

Amy Fadhli

Very few, if any, are born with perfect legs. Most people have to spend time shaping their legs into how they want them to look. The fitness stars spend a good deal of time working on their legs. Those who have awesome physiques – people like Mia Finnegan, Amy Fadhli, Monica Brant, Laurie Donnelly, Sherilyn Godreau, and many others take the time to work on their legs. They know that great legs don't come easily.

Can you change the appearance of your legs? Using specific training methods, you can change the shape of your legs. You were born with a certain leg structure, but you can alter the shape of your legs drastically. When it comes to the shape of your legs, you are not stuck with what you were born with – you can sculpt a new look if you know what to do and how to do it.

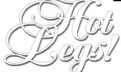

SHAPING A TIGHT & TRIM LOWER BODY

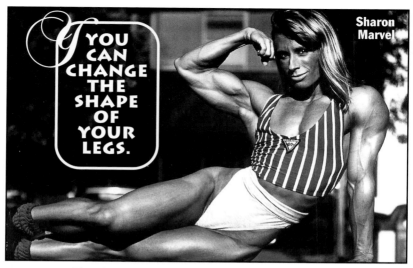

IF YOU CAN CHANGE THE SHAPE OF YOUR LEGS.

Sharon Marvel

Exercise is the best way to change the shape of your body. Tamilee Webb, (of *Buns of Steel* and *Abs of Steel* fame), was once teased about her body, but she used exercise to change the way she looked. Exercise can change your appearance significantly. That is where this book comes in. *Hot Legs!* will give you solid direction on how to shape, tighten and trim your lower body into the pair of hot legs you desire.

PRIMARY ELEMENTS

Changing the shape of the physique involves several elements. The physique can change for the worse, for instance, if it retains more fat. The body is comprised primarily of water, fat, muscle and bone. The bone structure is fairly well set by the time you become an adult, although you can make some changes by lifting weights and getting an adequate calcium intake. But these changes to the bone structure are fairly small. The two primary elements you have the ability to work with are changes in fat and muscle. By altering the amounts of fat and muscle in your physique, you can alter the shape of your body. For instance, if you don't exercise (and also tend to eat too much), you will lose muscle tone and strength, and you will accumulate fat. Your body will start to take on a more puffy appearance. On the other hand, if you begin to exercise on a consistent basis (and eat nutritiously), you will lose bodyfat, and increase your muscle tone and strength. Your legs will take on a more lean, tight, and shapely appearance. You can alter the shape of your legs – it is possible.

USE YOUR MIND AS WELL AS YOUR BODY TO TRAIN YOUR LEGS.

It is important to remember that there are two elements primarily responsible for the appearance of your legs – fat and muscle. It

SHAPING A TIGHT & TRIM LOWER BODY

Hot Legs!

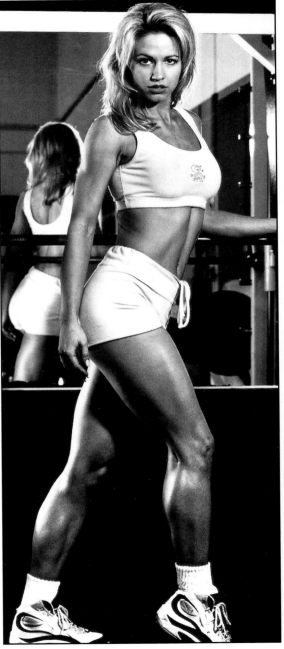

Brandy Hale

is crucial to know this in order to successfully shape you legs. Losing fat off of the legs is not enough. If you just lose fat and do not address the muscle, you will have trimmer legs, but they won't be tight – they will be small and loose instead of large and loose. To have hot legs you must work on the muscles. The opposite is also true. You cannot just work on the muscle tone and forget about the fat – then you will have legs that are tight, but not necessarily trim as they will be covered by a layer of fat. To create hot legs, you will have to focus on both elements – losing fat and adding muscle tone. How do you do that? To make serious change, you need the correct information and an organized plan. It is hard to get any solid growth from hit-and-miss effort.

This booklet will provide the information necessary to shape your legs properly, helping you aquire an impressively tight and trim appearance. The information will be set forth in an organized manner so that you can put it to work for your own purposes.

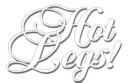

SHAPING A TIGHT & TRIM LOWER BODY

EFFORT

Shaping a pair of hot legs does not happen without a little effort on your part. The body does not willingly or easily change. It will resist your efforts to make it take on a new shape. But if your desire to change your legs is more than your desire to take it easy, you can accomplish what you want. You can make the shape and appearance of your legs change. A sculptor does not create a work of art without putting some effort forth – and the same is true for sculpting the shape of your legs. Effort is a required element which makes the change possible. You don't have to go overboard and overtrain your legs, but you will have to put in a good workout consistently.

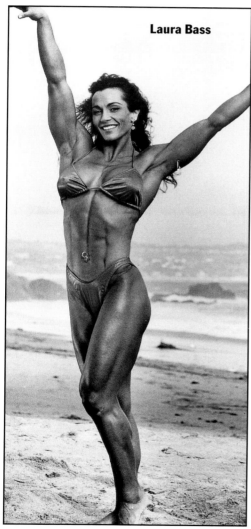

Laura Bass

CONSISTENCY

Another necessary ingredient in the *Hot Legs!* mix is consistency. Hit-and-miss workouts don't really add up to much. Consistency is crucial if you plan to change the shape of your physique. A physique shaping program must be consistent to expect change. The body does not easily change shape, and it is consistency that finally conquers it. Patient effort is a powerful tool when it comes to sculpting the legs. Although we live in an "instant" society, where everyone wants immediate action (for instance, the microwave, airplane, telephone, Internet, etc.), the body does not surrender its treasures quickly. You don't have to be a superstar to build great legs – you just have to be consistent in your workouts. Consistency is the great equalizer when it comes to training the body. Consistency means that you make it a habit to exercise your legs. You don't have to hit every workout flawlessly, but you do need to work your legs on a regular basis.

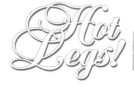

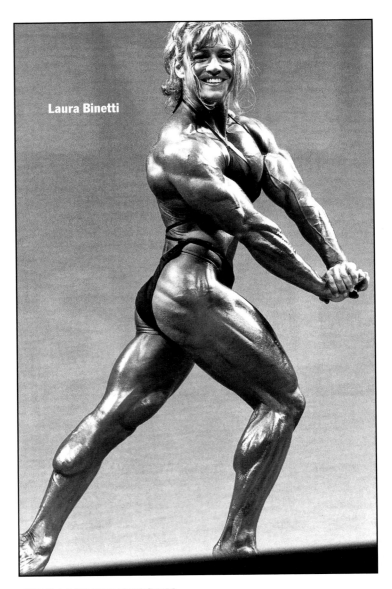

Laura Binetti

ORGANIZED EFFORT

You can work your legs in a haphazard manner and receive some gains. This is because your legs will respond to new stimuli, especially if they have not been trained previously. But your efforts will soon diminish if your workouts are not organized. You can get much better returns for your leg-training efforts if you have an organized plan. Intelligent, organized training is how you really force the body to progress.

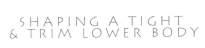

SHAPING A TIGHT
& TRIM LOWER BODY

So what do you do to get your leg-training efforts organized? If you want awesome looking legs, how do you get started? You could experiment by trial-and-error, but that takes a lot of time, and sometimes you don't draw the right conclusions from your training efforts. A better idea is to get some understanding of leg-training from fitness magazines and books. Best of all, *Hot Legs!* provides an organized approach to training the legs that is geared toward your needs. This booklet is specifically focused on one thing, leg-training. You don't need to use the trial-and-error method, or comb through dozens of magazines and books. Instead, you can take the quickest path to a pair of beautiful legs by using the material here. Of course, it is always good to use additional knowledge found in other articles, and trial-and-error adds to your learning process, but the shortest path to where you want to go is the *Hot Legs!* path. This book presents an organized process for shaping a beautifully contoured lower body. The workouts are custom-tailored to tone your legs, burn off unwanted fat, and increase muscle tissue, which will give your legs a firm, shapely appearance.

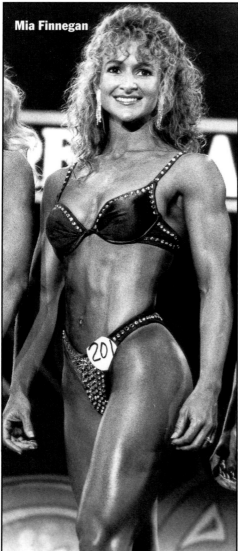

Mia Finnegan

The workout design of the *Hot Legs!* program is divided into distinct sections. First, an overview of training the largest leg area, the thighs (quadriceps), is presented. The preceding chapter focuses on the hamstrings (leg biceps), followed by a chapter on calf-training. Included is a chapter on the specific cardiovascular/ aerobic exercises that help tone the leg muscles while also burning off bodyfat to boot. Not all cardio/aerobic work utilizes the legs effec-

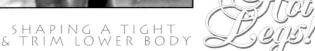

THE SHORTEST PATH TO A TIGHT AND TRIM LOWER BODY IS THE *HOT LEGS!* PATH.

tively enough to reshape them (some don't use the legs at all), so this chapter provides insight into the best cardio/aerobic exercises for the lower body. There is also a section in this booklet outlining a mixture of the various exercises, to provide a cohesive leg-training program. It is the combination of all the leg-training elements that will produce the greatest progress in your physique.

Use the insight and direction in this book to lead you on the path to a tighter and trimmer lower body. Take advantage of the material for the benefit of your legs. Read through each chapter until you grasp the leg-training concepts each chapter provides. Take some time getting to understand the various motions and mechanics of each exercise explained in the individual chapters, and the effect that each leg-training exercise is designed to have on your legs. Start to train your legs with your mind as well as your body. The mind is the most important and powerful "muscle" when it comes to training the body. The mind must lead the body for training to be fully effective. Your mind decides what your body is going to do, and then makes your body do it. For instance, fitness star Mia Finnegan dedicated almost as much time to mental preparation as she did to physical preparation in winning the top fitness title of Ms. Fitness Olympia (*Muscle & Fitness*, January 1996). So get tough mentally so that you can stick with your routine on a consistent basis.

If you consistently follow the training guidelines in the *Hot Legs!* program you should begin

A WELL-TRAINED PAIR OF LEGS PROVIDES NUMEROUS BENEFITS.

to notice a nice new shape to your legs, and the longer you stick with the *Hot Legs!* program, the more drastic and pronounced the changes will be. There are also other benefits that occur when you work your legs. Having a hot pair of "wheels" does more than just catch someone's eye. Well-trained legs are healthy legs, and healthy legs are a large part of a healthy body. Well-trained legs also provide you with an extra level of body strength, which is very beneficial, especially when you need to lift something or travel on foot somewhere.

Weight training will play a large role in shaping your legs. One of the first fitness stars, Rachel McLish, was a big proponent of weight training for shaping the legs. So was her predecessor, Cory Everson. The *Hot Legs!* program uses weight training combined with aerobic exercises and flexibility training, as will be described in the following pages.

Follow through with the training principles outlined in *Hot Legs!* and begin the process of reshaping your legs, as well as gaining an awesome feeling of health and vigor.

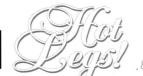

SHAPING A TIGHT & TRIM LOWER BODY

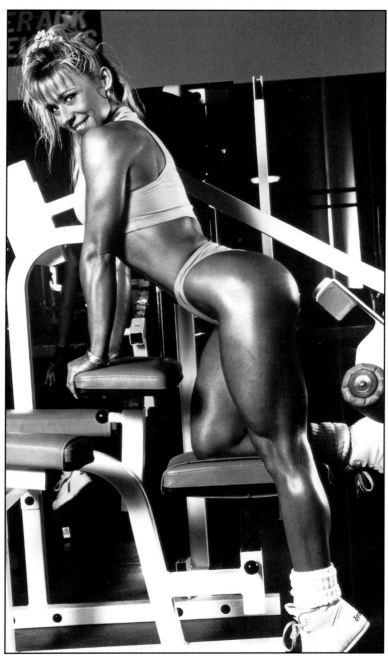

Pepper Ferry

Part Two
THE THIGHS

Your thighs, the frontal muscle group of your upper leg, are the biggest muscle group in your body. They are the strongest muscle group. A woman's thighs are surprisingly strong, even when compared to a man. Men are generally much stronger in the upper body, but there is a closer correlation with lower body strength. Since the thighs are such a major muscle group, it is important to train them right.

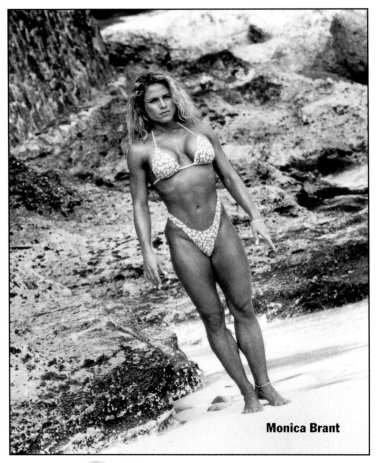

Monica Brant

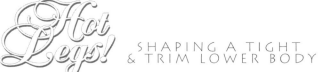

SHAPING A TIGHT
& TRIM LOWER BODY

The shape and condition of your thighs is a major factor in the appearance of your lower body. Thighs don't automatically look fantastic. They can be too large and fat, or too skinny and thin. Or they can be shaped oddly, (some are referred to as "turnip thighs," a condition where the upper thigh is too large in comparison to the lower thigh area). Since the thighs are such a major factor in the appearance of your legs, training them correctly becomes important.

YOU CAN ADD SHAPELY MUSCULARITY AND FIRMNESS TO YOUR LEGS WITH THE RIGHT TYPE OF TRAINING.

The goal of a good thigh-training program should be to build a pair of thighs that are tight, trim, and shapely. They should show some muscularity but not too much. The *Hot Legs!* thigh-training program is designed to achieve these goals – adding some muscularity and firmness without going too far. The exercises, especially those in the cardio/aerobic section, will also help burn off fat. The combination of adding shapely muscularity and firmness, along with losing fat, will produce an impressive looking pair of legs.

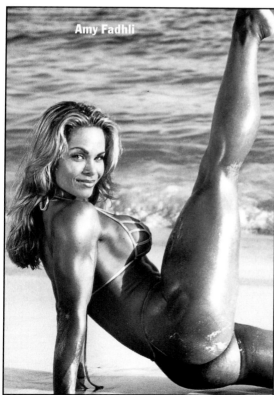
Amy Fadhli

WEIGHT TRAINING

The most rapid way in which to bring about change in your legs is with weight training. Fitness and bodybuilding star Sharon Bruneau related in *Muscle & Fitness* (August 1995) how weight training improved her shape and appearance. Weight training is the supreme manner in which to change your physique. When weight training is combined with a good cardio/aerobic routine that works the leg region, the changes to your legs can be awesome. Ms. Fitness World Carol Semple-Marzetta believes in a combination of weight training and cardio/aerobic work (*Muscle & Fitness*, November 1996). Cory Everson also believes in combining weight training and cardio/aerobic work for the best results, suggesting 30 minutes of resistance training followed by 30 minutes of cardio/aerobic work (*Muscle & Fitness*, November 1996). The combination is dynamic.

Weight training progressively challenges your body (and your legs in particular) to higher levels of change through an increasingly difficult stimulus. Your body responds to the new demands by

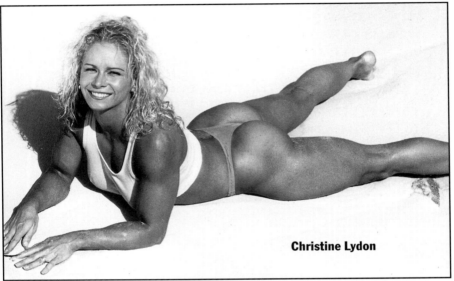

Christine Lydon

becoming firmer, more muscular, and less fat. These dynamics of weight training can be successfully applied to your legs to make them change for the better. All you need to do is follow some basic principles that make weight training successful in shaping your body. These essential principles include consistency, following good form when you lift, and (especially) progressive resistance.

> **THE SINGLE MOST EFFECTIVE MANNER IN WHICH TO CHANGE YOUR LEGS IS THROUGH WEIGHT TRAINING.**

Weight training makes your muscles grow and this in turn helps you become tighter and trimmer. Fitness star Marjo Selin points out that "scientists have shown that every pound of muscle you add to your body requires an additional 50 to 100 calories a day to function. In other words, your caloric maintenance levels go up. This promotes using stored bodyfat for energy" (*MuscleMag International*, May 1988). When you add some muscle to your body, then your metabolic rate goes up and you burn off more bodyfat, even when in a resting state. This is one of the many benefits of weight training.

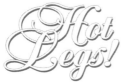

PROGRESSIVE RESISTANCE

Progressive resistance is crucial to your weight-training program because once your body has become accustomed to the workload you have presented it with, it ceases to gain and slips into a maintenance mode. This is fine if you just want to maintain your current condition, but if you want to improve you will need to take your training up to another level. For example, if you are using 50 pounds in a weight-training exercise for your legs, you will experience some positive physical changes. But if you use the 50-pound weight for the same amount of sets and repetitions each week (a set is a group of repetitions; a repetition is one full movement of the exercise) your body will not respond to the challenge of lifting 50 pounds any further. It will maintain the level it is at, but it will not go beyond that level. To step back into the growth mode you will need to increase the amount of weight you are using. If you had been using 50 pounds for a couple of sets of 15 repetitions and had been doing this for quite some time, you would want to increase the amount of weight you use to perhaps 60 pounds. Initially this increase in weight will lower the amount of repetitions you can perform in good form. You might be able to only perform 8 repetitions. But as you continue to use the heavier weight over the next few weeks, your body will gradually adjust to the new challenge, and you will eventually be able to lift the heavier weight for as many as 15 repetitions. This progression is how you challenge your body to improve on a consistent basis.

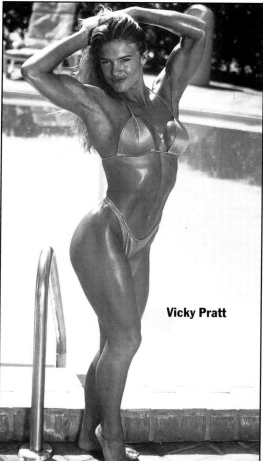

Vicky Pratt

FORM

Good form is also an essential element of successful lifting. You want the muscle you are focusing on to do the work, not other muscles. This means no

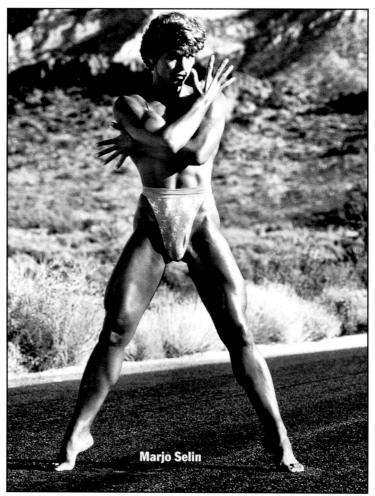
Marjo Selin

"cheating" to lift the weight. Paying close attention to good form is crucial. One writer who watched two fitness stars (Marla Duncan and Debbie Kruck) work out noted that they used excellent form. Jackie Paisley pointed out that she does her sets extra strict, slow, and makes sure she is getting the full range of movement (*Flex*, August 1990). That is what good form is all about.

REST AND RECUPERATION

Vital to your body's response to the challenges of weight training is adequate rest and recuperation. Rest and recuperation are essential for your body to add firmness and shapely muscle. The body does not grow or change when you workout! It only grows and changes while you rest and sleep. Adequate nutrition,

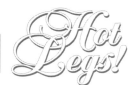

SHAPING A TIGHT
& TRIM LOWER BODY

sleep, rest, and recuperation are essential if you are to make positive physical changes to your body. The best rule of thumb for R & R is to give each major muscle group you train at least 48 to 72 hours of rest between workouts. This means taking two or three days off before you work the same muscle group again. If you work a major muscle group every day you will soon become overtrained and lose any previous muscle gains. The body needs rest and recuperation, particularly when it is in the middle of a training program.

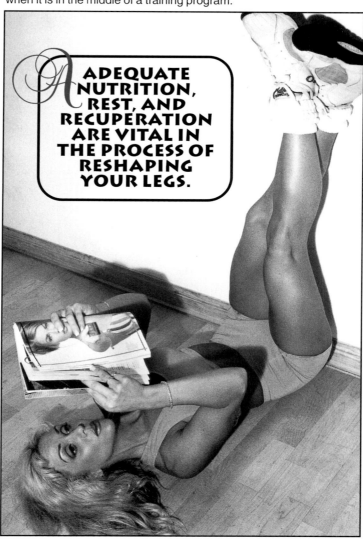

ADEQUATE NUTRITION, REST, AND RECUPERATION ARE VITAL IN THE PROCESS OF RESHAPING YOUR LEGS.

Leigh Anne Ross

GOOD TRAINING FORM FOCUSES THE EFFECT OF WEIGHT TRAINING ON YOUR SPECIFIC TARGET.

Good form when weight training is important because the better your training form, the better you can focus its effects on the area you want to change. Good training form also prevents injury to the body, which is very important when training the muscles of the legs.

In conclusion, when training the thighs you will need to use weight training on a consistent basis in good form; you will need to approach weight training in a progressive manner; and you will need to give the thighs some rest and recuperation between workouts. If you adhere to these guidelines you can really change the shape of your legs.

Debra Kaniho performs Smith machine squats in perfect form.

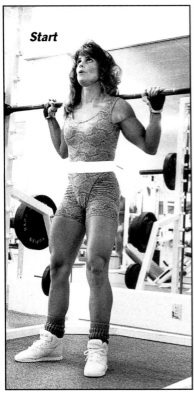

Start

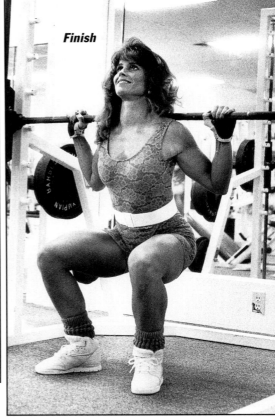

Finish

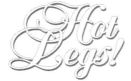

SHAPING A TIGHT & TRIM LOWER BODY

THE THIGH EXERCISES

There are several exercises that work well for shaping the thighs. These exercises will be described so that you can get a good grasp on how to attain trim and tight thighs – legs that demand a second look!

THE SQUAT

The squat is probably the best known leg exercise, and with good reason. It is the best way to work the total thigh muscle. The squat is legendary for changing the shape of thousands of legs. For example, two women with awesome legs, Tonya Knight and Marjo Selin, are often seen in fitness magazines using the squat to shape their legs. The squat is performed exactly as it sounds. You place a barbell across your upper back, and slowly squat down until your thighs are level with the ground. This position looks as if you are sitting on air. You then slowly stand up to a fully extended position.

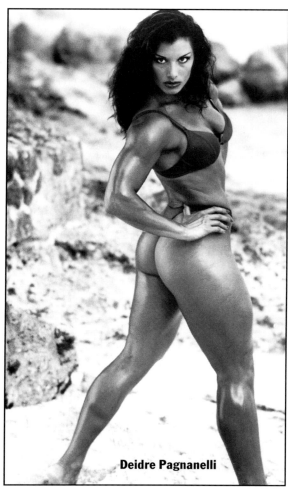

Deidre Pagnanelli

Practice this movement with only a bar across your back to get into the groove of the motion. Make sure to keep your shoulders and your back as straight as possible.

The squat is a tough movement to perform but it is necessary. The squat really works the deep fibers of the thigh muscles. When you use the squat movement, you can elevate your feet by placing a block or other solid object under your heels if you choose (make certain the object is stationary and won't flip up when you stand on it). Take a narrow stance (feet approximately shoulder-width apart) and keep your head and chest up. Keeping your head and chest up and taking a narrow stance all work together to put the stress of the movement on your thighs instead of your hips and buttocks. It is good to squat in this manner to avoid making the hips and buttocks grow. A wide stance with flat feet tends to put the emphasis on the gluteus maximus, which is fine if you are trying to build up your buttocks, but not if you are trying to keep your backside trim. So use a narrow stance, elevate your heels a couple of inches and keep your head and chest up.

A couple of sets of 8 to 10 repetitions works well for the squat. However, perform a warmup set or two with very light weight at first to loosen up the knee joints. To really get some strength and shape into your legs, try an occasional set of 20 repetitions. This high-repetition range will really push your legs to a new level of development. The squat is a great thigh builder if you use it right.

THE SISSY SQUAT

The sissy squat is another fantastic thigh exercise. This exercise is tagged the "sissy" squat because it is often performed without weight. It looks like it is easier than the regular squat, but it isn't! When performed correctly, the sissy squat really gives the middle thigh a burn. The sissy squat works the long muscles of the leg, the muscles that run from the hip down to the knee, in an arch. This muscle group, when developed, really adds to the beauty

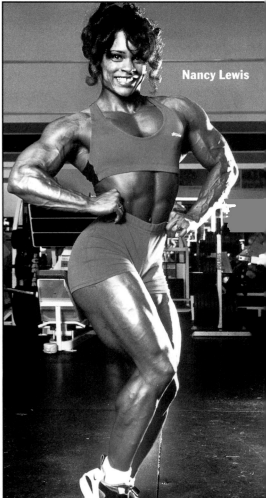

Nancy Lewis

of the thigh. It builds the thigh up in the middle area, and also ties in the entire musculature of the upper leg. When the sissy squat is used regularly, the leg muscles develop in such a manner as to give the illusion of the legs being longer than they really are. Dayna Albrecht knows what sissy squats are capable of producing – beautiful, trim legs – so she uses 4 sets of sissy squats in her leg routine (*MuscleMag International*, April 1995).

The sissy squat is performed by standing with your heels on an elevated surface. Squat down, but squat with a forward thrust of the hips

THE SISSY SQUAT, WHEN USED OFTEN, CREATES A BEAUTIFUL PAIR OF LEGS.

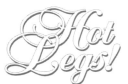

SHAPING A TIGHT & TRIM LOWER BODY

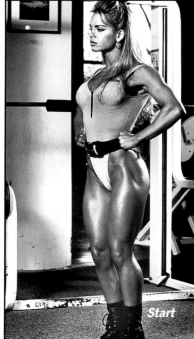
Start

as you go down. Your knees will travel forward, and your legs will arch outward. When you get as far forward and down as possible, drop your hips until they almost touch the ground. From this position reverse the action, pushing your hips forward, and standing back up in the arched leg manner. The use of these unique movements and angles places the stress of the movement on the middle and long muscles of the leg, creating a stimulus for these areas to respond. As your legs respond to the training challenge that the sissy squat provides, they will really start to develop a fabulous appearance. Once you have mastered this movement without weight you can place a light barbell across your upper chest to add resistance.

ROMAN-CHAIR SQUATS

This exercise sounds nasty, but it produces beautiful legs, so it is well worth the effort. To perform this exercise you will need a Roman-chair squat machine. Some gyms have these; if not, they can be ordered from various weight-training companies. This exercise is performed by squatting backward and letting the machine hold your lower legs in place. Put your hands at your side, and sit down into a low position, then stand back up, but not all of the way. Do not allow the knees to lock as this will keep sufficient stress on the leg muscles, helping to shape and firm them quicker.

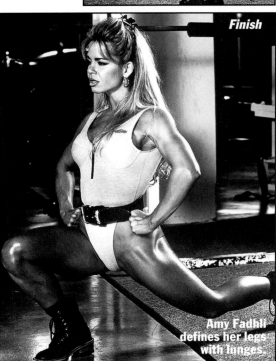
Finish

Amy Fadhli defines her legs with lunges.

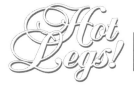

SHAPING A TIGHT & TRIM LOWER BODY

THE LUNGE

The lunge is a good exercise for adding nice definition (lines in the legs) to the thighs. This exercise is performed by placing a light barbell across your back, then "lunging" slowly forward on one foot, keeping the other leg stationary. Push yourself back to the starting position using the thigh muscles, then perform the same movement but with the opposite leg. Keep your balance, and make the thighs do all of the work. Ms. Olympia, Lenda Murray, points out in a *Flex* article (November 1995) that the lunge is great for firming up the lower body. Nikki Fuller does an interesting variation of the lunge, called walking lunges, performing them for 50 to 100 meters nonstop (*Flex*, January 1993).

THE HACK SQUAT IS PROBABLY THE BEST "MACHINE" EXERCISE FOR THE THIGHS.

THE HACK SQUAT

The hack squat is a fantastic exercise; it may be the best leg-machine exercise available. It gives a wonderful outer sweep to the thighs. Step into the hack-squat machine and place your feet in a relatively narrow position (closer than shoulder width). Keep your back straight and your head

Start

Finish

Use a high-repetition range when performing the leg extension.
– Coralie Mosby

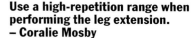

SHAPING A TIGHT & TRIM LOWER BODY

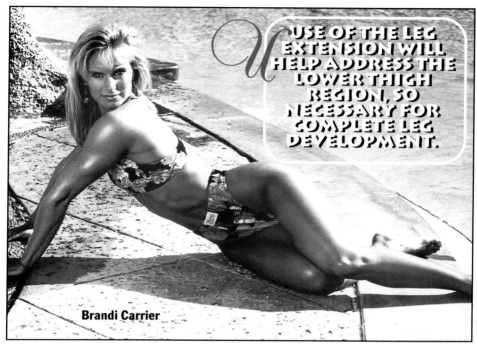

USE OF THE LEG EXTENSION WILL HELP ADDRESS THE LOWER THIGH REGION, SO NECESSARY FOR COMPLETE LEG DEVELOPMENT.

Brandi Carrier

up, and lower your body all of the way, then up again. The hack squat is great because it forces the right muscles (the lower and outer thigh areas) to perform the work. These lower and outer thigh muscles look great when developed. Rene Redden uses the hack squat for 3 sets of 15 repetitions in one of her leg-training cycles (*Ironman*, February 1996).

THE LEG EXTENSION

Another very good machine exercise for the thighs is the leg extension. The leg extension primarily works the lower muscles of the thigh, right above the knee area. This area is important to develop because a large upper thigh without adequate lower thigh development distorts the appearance of the leg, giving it the "turnip" look. How do you overcome this thigh appearance problem? The hack squat helps, but the leg extension is especially helpful for doing away with the "turnip" look. When you perform the leg extension, never let the legs rest. Lock the weight out at the top of the position, and squeeze the lower thigh muscles hard for a full second. Use a high-repetition range for the leg-extension movement. Sandy Riddell uses the leg extension for thigh shape, separation, and definition (*MuscleMag International*, October 1988). Dale Tomita also uses several sets of leg extensions in her leg-training routine (*Ironman*, February 1997).

THE THIGH WORKOUT

The exercises highlighted in this chapter are the best for shaping awesome thighs. These exercises can be used individually, but when you combine them into a full workout program they work even better. A few thigh-training routines are put together to provide you with an idea on how to use them to build hot legs!

> **ALTERNATING THIGH EXERCISES IS GOOD FOR THE MUSCLES, AS YOU WANT TO HIT THE ENTIRE LEG, AND GOOD FOR THE MIND, ELIMINATING THE POSSIBILITY OF BOREDOM.**

It is unwise to use all of the thigh exercises in each workout – remember, you still have hamstrings and calves to train. A couple of thigh exercises per workout will be enough. You have more than one exercise to choose

Dale Tomita

from. This eliminates the possibility of training boredom. Alternating thigh exercises, or any exercises, is good for the muscles, and prevents you from getting into a training rut. Variety is good for the mind and the muscles. The groupings of these exercises is by no means hard and fast. If you find a different set-up works better for you, by all means use what you come up with. But by planning your workout routine around these excellent exercises, you won't go wrong.

These are just a few of the many combinations available for working on the thighs in a way that shapes and firms up the muscularity in an appealing and symmetrical manner. If you feel you are

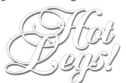

Hot Legs!

SHAPING A TIGHT
& TRIM LOWER BODY

THIGH-TRAINING ROUTINES

WORKOUT 1

Exercise	Sets	Repetitions
Squats	2	8-10
Sissy Squats	2	10-15

WORKOUT 2

Exercise	Sets	Repetitions
Squats	2	8-10
Leg Extensions	2	10-15

WORKOUT 3

Exercise	Sets	Repetitions
Hack Squats	2	8-12
Roman-chair Squats	2	10-15

WORKOUT 4

Exercise	Sets	Repetitions
Leg Extensions	2	10-15
Lunges	2	10-15

WORKOUT 5

Exercise	Sets	Repetitions
High-rep Squats	2	20
Roman-chair Squats	2	10-15

WORKOUT 6

Exercise	Sets	Repetitions
Leg Extensions	3	10-12
Sissy Squats	2	10-15

not receiving enough stimulation with 2 sets per exercise you can go up to 3 or even 4 sets per exercise. However, remember that you will also be performing work on your hamstrings and calves, so don't use all of your energy on your frontal thighs and have nothing left to use on the rest of your leg workout. When you train the thighs, use enough weight for each exercise so that the last couple of repetitions are quite difficult, but enable you to use good form.

These exercises work the upper leg in a thorough manner, especially if you use an adequate amount of weight. These exercises will help you make your thighs a contributing part of your hot legs! But the thigh is only one part of the leg, and only covers the front half. The back of the leg, the hamstring, is a muscle group that can also look absolutely fantastic if developed correctly. Part three focuses on the hamstrings, and how to make them contribute to your hot legs!

SHAPING A TIGHT
& TRIM LOWER BODY

Part Three
THE HAMSTRINGS

Your thighs are your largest leg muscles, however, your hamstrings may be your most beautiful muscles. The hamstring muscles, when sufficiently developed, form an attractive arch of muscle from just below your buttocks to just above the back of your knee. When this area is not developed it is either flat and non-descriptive (translated – boring), or it is flabby. On the other side of the coin, however, is the fact that well-developed hamstrings are a major part of having amazing legs. They make the legs look fantastic when they are firmed up. To realize the vast potential your hamstrings have for drastically changing the appearance of your legs, you will need to work on them with specific exercises. *Hot Legs!* will provide you with the necessary information to transform the look and fitness of the rear part of your legs, the hamstrings.

THE HAMSTRINGS CAN BE DEVELOPED SO AS TO BECOME YOUR MOST ATTRACTIVE LEG MUSCLES.

The chief function of the hamstrings is to pull your feet upward; the hamstring also acts as a brake on the leg as it descends. The squat movement, which figures so prominently in developing the thighs, uses the hamstring muscles only minimally. Other exercises are needed to really work the hamstrings. There are two exercise styles that really focus on working the hamstring muscles – leg-curl movements, and the stiff-leg deadlift movement. Both should be incorporated into your leg-

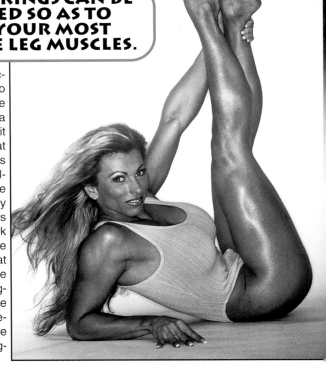

Stacey Lynn

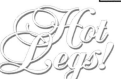

SHAPING A TIGHT
& TRIM LOWER BODY

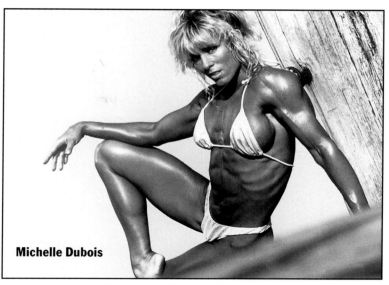

Michelle Dubois

training program. Fitness star Rene Redden uses 3 sets of each when training her legs (*Ironman*, February 1996).

LEG CURLS

Leg curls are perhaps the most well-known exercise for the hamstring muscles. A machine has been specifically built for working the hamstring muscle group. This machine, the leg-curl machine, consists of a padded bench, a stack of attached weights, and an attached

> **USE A SLOW AND STEADY PACE WHEN PERFORMING THE LEG-CURL MOVEMENT.**

padded bar. You lie in a face-down position and put the back of your feet under the padded bar at the rear of the machine. From this position you curl your feet towards your buttocks against the resistance of the padded bar (which is attached to the weight stack). This motion really engages the hamstring muscles, which put forth the primary effort in the pulling motion.

When performing the leg curl from the prone position, let your legs extend all of the way to the bottom (slowly), then smoothly curl them towards your buttocks. Stop the motion just before you reach the top (when your feet are just above your buttocks), keeping the tension on your hamstrings. Do not let the padded bar bounce into your buttocks or become slack – keep a slow, steady tension on the hamstrings. Do not use explosive action for the leg-curl movement. Keep all leg-curling motions slow and steady. If you use explosive movements during the leg-curl exercise you may injure your hamstring muscles. You also remove the pressure from the muscle at the top and bottom of the movement, decreasing the effectiveness of the exercise. You can feel the hamstring muscles as they work – there is significant pressure in that region of the leg, to know when the focus is on the muscle and when it is not. Your aim is to keep the pressure on the hamstrings during the entire leg-curling motion. Sure, it is somewhat painful, especially during the last few repetitions, but this pain (it should be a slight pain – stop if it starts to become too sharp) will develop the firmness in the leg you desire. You can help keep the pressure on the hamstrings during this exercise by leaning on your elbows.

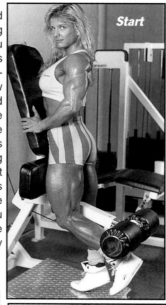

Start

KEEP THE PRESSURE ON THE HAMSTRING MUSCLES CONSTANT THROUGHOUT THE ENTIRE LEG-CURL MOVEMENT.

Use a moderately high-repetition range for the hamstring muscles. This means 8 to 15 repetitions, with the last 2 to 3 repetitions being fairly tough to complete. When you can perform 10 to 15 repetitions easily it is time to increase the weight resistance.

Another version of the leg-curl movement is the standing leg-curl exercise. Instead of lying in a prone position, you stand on one foot, with the other foot hooked into the standing leg-curl machine. You curl the padded bar toward the buttocks as with the

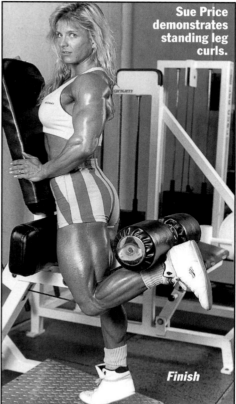

Sue Price demonstrates standing leg curls.

Finish

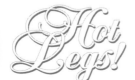

SHAPING A TIGHT & TRIM LOWER BODY

prone position. The motion for the standing leg curl is very similar to the prone leg curl, except that you are upright. This upright position is more helpful in keeping the pressure on the back of the legs as gravity assists in the action.

A variation of this version of the leg curl (the standing leg curl) can be performed with a cable machine if you have a foot attachment. Secure the attachment to your ankle, with the front hook on the front of your foot. Attach the hook to a cable-pulley weight stack, and curl your leg backward.

Yet another version of the leg curl is to attach a weight to your ankle (with something such as a weighted strap, etc.) and then curl your foot toward your buttocks. Since most weighted leg straps are fairly light, increase the repetitions (up to 25+) as you become accustomed to this exercise.

STIFF-LEG DEADLIFTS

Not everyone has access to the various leg-curling exercise machines; however, this doesn't give you adequate reason to skip hamstring workouts. The hamstrings need to be worked if you want hot legs! There is no need to worry if you cannot get the equipment to perform the leg curl. The best hamstring exercise can be performed with just a barbell. The very best hamstring exercise is the stiff-leg

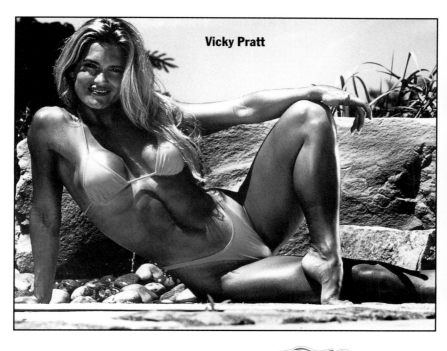

Vicky Pratt

deadlift. The stiff-leg deadlift uses the hamstring muscles as the primary levers in the performance of lifting the weight upward. This exercise is performed by holding a barbell at waist level, using a shoulder-width grip. While keeping the legs straight, bend forward until your upper body is almost parallel with the

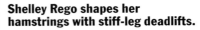

ONE OF THE VERY BEST HAMSTRING EXERCISES IS THE STIFF-LEG DEADLIFT.

floor. Only the upper body moves as the hip area acts like a hinge. The arms should also be kept straight and fairly loose throughout the entire movement. Use a light weight, particularly in the initial stages. As you lower yourself down (keeping your back very straight), keep your head up, looking at the top of the nearest wall. Only go down far enough so that the barbell is level with your upper shins (do not let the barbell get near to touching the ground). When the barbell is at the level of your upper shins, come back to an upright position. This constitutes one repetition. You will really feel the hamstrings work in this exercise if you perform it in strict fashion. As with the leg curl, use a moderately high-repetition range (8 to 15 repetitions).

Shelley Rego shapes her hamstrings with stiff-leg deadlifts.

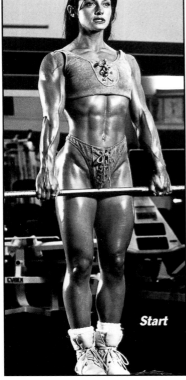

Start

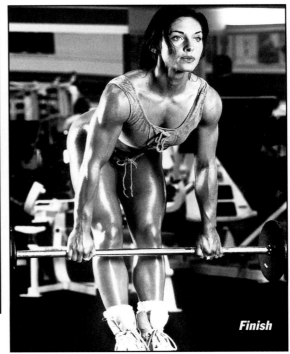

Finish

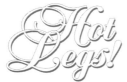

SHAPING A TIGHT & TRIM LOWER BODY

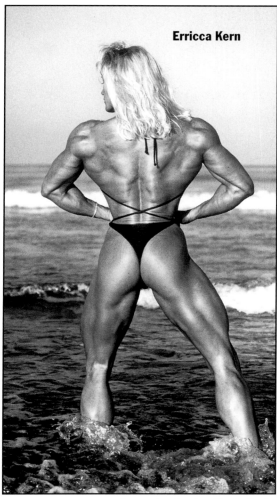

Erricca Kern

The stiff-leg deadlift exercise can also be performed with dumbells if you do not have (or have access to) a barbell.

To speed up the process of your hamstring-training you can perform some flexing and contracting motions for the hamstring muscles. These motions are performed "freestyle," that is, without weight. You plant your bodyweight on one leg, putting the ball of your other foot on some type of a ledge (such as the horizontal leg of a bench, or a low step). Pull with your bent leg. Pull as hard as you can for a few seconds, then let your foot come free and slowly bring it up to your buttocks. Repeat a few times with each leg.

Stretching is also important for good hamstring development. Stretch your hamstrings before, during, and after your workouts. Spend a few minutes getting a good relaxing stretch, then push yourself, as you progress, to stretch a little more. Stretching really helps shape the legs, and goes hand-in-hand with weight training.

A couple of sets of both the leg curl and the stiff-leg deadlift per workout will really start to shape your hamstrings nicely. If you do not have access to a leg-curl apparatus, then perform 3 sets of the stiff-leg deadlift. These hamstring exercises should be mixed in with the thigh exercises, working your full legs in one routine. An overall integrated leg-training routine is included in part five of *Hot Legs!*

STRETCHING WILL REALLY ASSIST IN THE DEVELOPMENT AND SHAPE OF YOUR HAMSTRING MUSCLES.

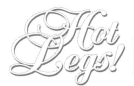

Part Four
THE CALF WORKOUT

The hamstrings have been noted as a beautiful muscle group when they are fully developed but they have a major contender – the calves. The calves are the major muscle group of the lower leg, and also the most visible of all the leg-muscle groups. You might be able to hide your upper legs some of the time, but you cannot get away with hiding your calves for long. For this reason, it makes sense to develop your calf muscles. As with the other muscle groups, the calves can be developed to look much more attractive – if you have the desire, put forth the effort, and do so consistently. The calves play a major role in hot legs! This chapter will give you some ideas on shaping your calves.

The primary function of the calf muscle is to push your body upward, and onward. They play a major role in walking. You can feel your calves work if you stand on your toes.

In order for the calves to change, they need to get a full extension – in both directions. They need to be able to extend down as far as possible, and also to be able to go up as far as possible. Half extensions, or extensions in only one direction, do not develop the calf

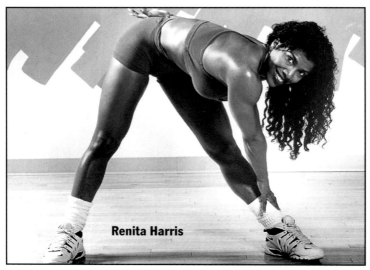

Renita Harris

Hot Legs!
SHAPING A TIGHT
& TRIM LOWER BODY

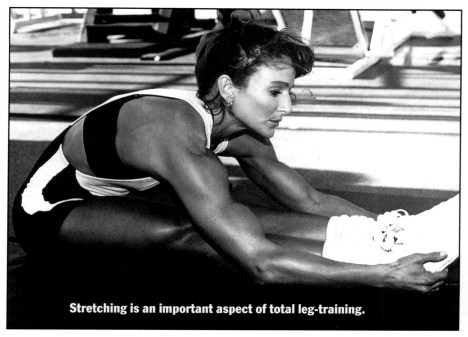

Stretching is an important aspect of total leg-training.

muscle to its full potential. The heel needs to go below the horizontal plane on the downstroke of a calf exercise, and it needs to extend far above the horizontal plane on the upstroke of an exercise. When it is allowed to be exercised in this fashion full development can occur, particularly when the exercise involves increasing challenges. The calf muscle, when developed, becomes firm, shapely, and very appealing to the eye.

> **STRETCHING THE CALVES ON A REGULAR BASIS WILL GREATLY ASSIST IN THEIR DEVELOPMENT.**

STRETCHING

Before you get started using exercises to build up your calves it is a good idea to spend some time stretching your calf muscles. One of the best ways to do this is by putting the ball and toe area of one foot on a raised surface (such as a step) and pushing your heel down. Hold this position for several seconds, then switch to the other calf. Work at this for a few days until you can stretch each calf for longer than one minute. Also stretch the calf in the reverse manner, standing on the step with your heel and pointing your toes upward.

After a few days of stretching move on to some freestyle calf exercises. These can be performed on a step. Stand with your heels off the step, and the balls of your feet on the step. Balance yourself and lower the calves all the way down

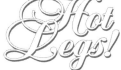

(use a step that is high enough to let you fully extend your heels without touching the floor), then push yourself back up, fully extending the calf. Perform several repetitions and a few sets for each foot.

WEIGHT-TRAINED CALVES

The calves can be a difficult and challenging muscle group to get a response from. The larger leg muscles seem to readily respond in comparison to training the calves. This is a general statement – a few people have calves that respond immediately, but most have to really work the calves to get some change. The best way to stimulate the calves to new firmness and shape is with weight training. Fitness star Marla Duncan points out in *Ironman* (October 1994) that she trains her calves every day. Weight training is a super manner in which to shape any part of the body, and calf-training is no exception. The following are several effective weight-training movements that can be used to shape and firm the calf muscles.

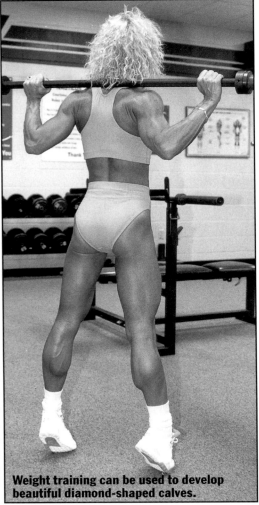

Weight training can be used to develop beautiful diamond-shaped calves.

DUMBELL CALF RAISES

The dumbell calf raise is a simple exercise easily performed at home with only a dumbell and a step. It is essentially the same exercise as the freestyle calf raise mentioned earlier, but with the added resistance of a dumbell. You stand on a step with one foot, putting

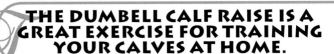

THE DUMBELL CALF RAISE IS A GREAT EXERCISE FOR TRAINING YOUR CALVES AT HOME.

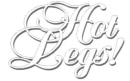

your weight on the ball of the foot and letting the heel hang free. Balance yourself with one hand, and hold the dumbell in the other (a light dumbell initially). Go all of the way down and up on one foot, slow and steady. Make sure to "feel" the calf muscle as it works. Get a full extension on both the downward and upward motions of the movement. Perform several repetitions – enough so your calf muscle starts to "burn" with muscle-effort pain, then switch to the other foot. Perform 2 to 5 sets of this exercise for each calf if it is the only calf exercise in your routine. (This is particularly applicable to those who train at home.)

SEATED CALF RAISES

A fantastic exercise for developing the calves is the seated calf raise. The seated calf raise is performed on a seated calf-raise machine. Most gyms and fitness centers have at least one of these machines, and they also can be bought through mail-order companies, which often advertise in fitness magazines. If you have some extra space such as in the garage or a spare room you might consider obtaining your own calf machine. The seated calf-raise machine places direct pressure on the calf muscles. You place your knees under a padded bar, and place the balls of your feet on the lower bar of the machine. You lift the weight in a similar motion to the other calf exercises mentioned, extending slowly down, then up. The pressure on a seated-calf machine is supplied by the weight on the vertical bar at the end of the machine. This weight is

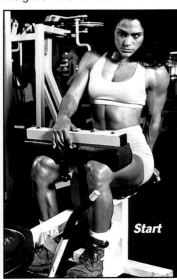

Start

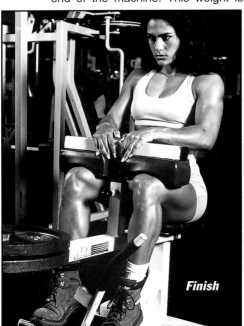

Finish

Michelle Greer works her calves with seated calf-raises.

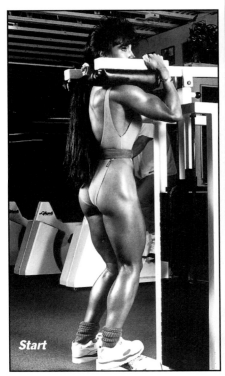

Start

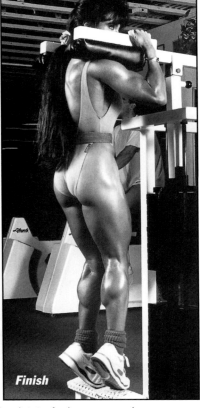

Finish

Lisa Lorio pumps her calves with standing calf raises.

leveraged weight, so you will not need a lot to feel your muscles working. Experiment with the weight until you reach an amount that makes the last few repetitions of each set difficult to perform.

STANDING CALF RAISES

The standing calf raise is similar to the freestyle calf raise. With the standing calf raise there are a couple of differences – it is performed on an apparatus that has weights attached, and you use both feet instead of one. This allows you to use more weight. It is a good idea to use lighter weight at first though, to become accustomed to the movement. Make sure to keep your body straight as you perform the movement to keep the emphasis on the calf muscles. Get a good full stretch for maximum benefit.

FLEXING AND STRETCHING

As you work on the calf muscles, spend a good amount of time and effort flexing and stretching them. Tighten and relax the calf muscles frequently. Stretch the calf muscles between each set of the calf workout, and also before and after the workout.

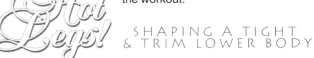

SHAPING A TIGHT
& TRIM LOWER BODY

SETS AND REPETITIONS

The calf muscles are dense muscles and generally need more work than the upper leg muscles. This translates into a higher repetition range (12 to 20) and more sets. You can also assist the process by taking less rest between sets when you work on the calf muscles, which keep the muscles pumped and tight. Less time between sets makes the calves work harder and grow quicker. With most of the larger muscle groups you want to take more rest between sets, but the calves are different and can handle a quicker paced workout, so don't "baby" them.

The calf workouts can be integrated into the full leg workout, or they can be performed on separate days. A few examples of the integrated approach (mixing calf work with upper leg exercises) will be noted later. You should perform at least a few sets of calf work every few days.

The calf muscles can be trained and shaped to have a firm and more attractive appearance. They are one of the most visible lower body muscles, so if you want hot legs you need to put some time and effort into your calves. Diamond-shaped calves don't have to be a dream. Work hard and you'll see the results.

Marjo Selin

> A HIGH-REPETITION RANGE AND MORE SETS GENERALLY WORKS BEST WHEN TRAINING THE CALVES.

Part Five
CARDIO/AEROBIC
CONNECTION

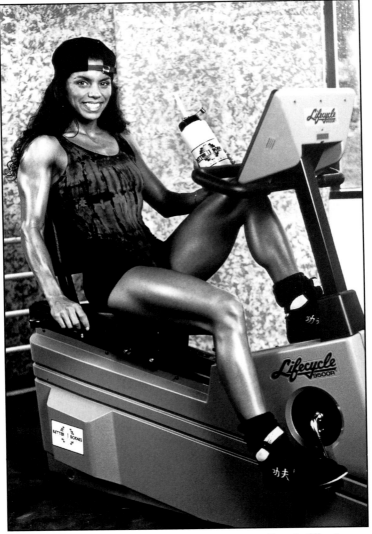

Ursula Alberto

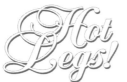
Hot Legs!

SHAPING A TIGHT
& TRIM LOWER BODY

There is a large variety of cardiovascular/aerobic exercises that are used by people to get in shape. Up to this point in the *Hot Legs!* program the focus has been on the anaerobic exercises – the working of the muscles in brief, intense and concentrated motions with weights. However, there is also a connection between cardiovascular/aerobic work and the legs. Some of the wide variety

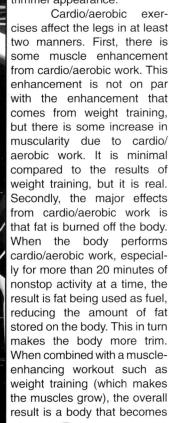

of cardio/aerobic exercises affect the legs. On the other side of the coin, some do not. For instance, the rowing exercise primarily affects the upper body as the legs are held stationary during this movement. Part five of *Hot Legs!* will focus on how certain cardio/aerobic exercises can help you in shaping your legs to attain a tighter and trimmer appearance.

Cardio/aerobic exercises affect the legs in at least two manners. First, there is some muscle enhancement from cardio/aerobic work. This enhancement is not on par with the enhancement that comes from weight training, but there is some increase in muscularity due to cardio/ aerobic work. It is minimal compared to the results of weight training, but it is real. Secondly, the major effects from cardio/aerobic work is that fat is burned off the body. When the body performs cardio/aerobic work, especially for more than 20 minutes of nonstop activity at a time, the result is fat being used as fuel, reducing the amount of fat stored on the body. This in turn makes the body more trim. When combined with a muscle-enhancing workout such as weight training (which makes the muscles grow), the overall result is a body that becomes

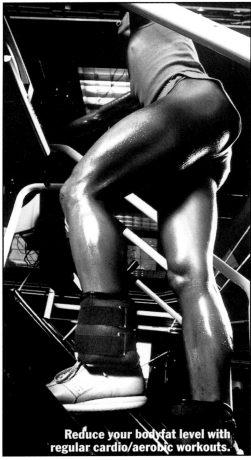

Reduce your body fat level with regular cardio/aerobic workouts.

SHAPING A TIGHT
& TRIM LOWER BODY

tighter and trimmer. That is the goal of the *Hot Legs!* program – to shape a tighter and trimmer lower body. Another benefit acquired from more muscle and less fat is a faster metabolism, which burns off even more fat.

Several exercises work well for getting a combination effect from cardio/aerobic exercise. A few of the better ones will be highlighted in this chapter.

STAIR STEPPING

Stair stepping is an excellent way to get a great cardio/aerobic workout, while placing most of the emphasis on the legs. Stair stepping gives the legs a constant challenge and they readily respond by

becoming tighter and trimmer. Muscularity increases while fat decreases when you use the stair stepper. There are a variety of stair-stepping machines available. Most gyms have several. You can also obtain a home unit, and there is even a very small unit suitable for traveling. However, machine stair stepping is not the only possibility. You can climb stairs – real stairs – if you have access to them. Whatever type of stair stepping you choose to use for your workout, make certain your workouts last for more than 20 minutes (after your first few initial workouts which may be less than 20 minutes as you become accustomed to the workout). A 30- to 45-minute stair-stepping workout is fantastic for your legs and also burns off a lot of fat – fat that is not just on your legs, but all over your body. A few stair stepping workouts per week will

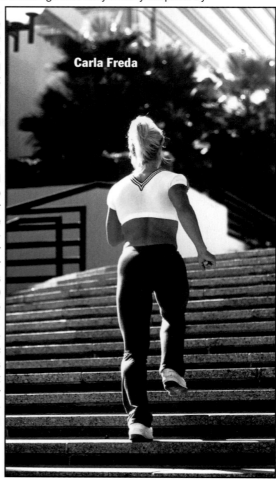

Carla Freda

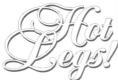

SHAPING A TIGHT
& TRIM LOWER BODY

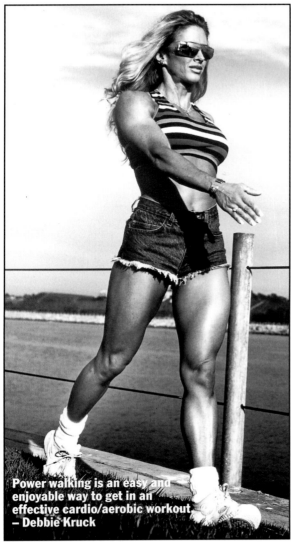

Power walking is an easy and enjoyable way to get in an effective cardio/aerobic workout.
— Debbie Kruck

really start to shape your legs if you are consistent with your workouts.

POWER WALKING

Power walking is another great exercise for the legs. Power walking also places all of the emphasis on the legs as the primary tool for movement. Power walking should be performed at a pace that is quite brisk and at a continuous rate. Walk as fast as you can, getting a good push-off on each step and consciously tightening the buttocks as you walk. After a few initial walks, aim at power walking for 30 to 45 minutes per session. If you can take an occasional walk that is longer than this do so. Power walking can be performed outdoors or indoors – but most people like to get out and go for a refreshing walk.

It is not always possible to go outdoors for a power walk; therefore, the treadmill is a good alternative. Fitness star Cameo Kneuer relates in *Muscle & Fitness* (October 1994) that she uses both brisk walking and the treadmill. The treadmill allows you to walk indoors during nasty weather which would otherwise curtail your routine, and it allows you to get in a full workout in a limited space. Most gyms and fitness centers have several treadmills available, and they can be purchased fairly inexpensively. A further enhancement to the caloric burning potential is that many treadmills can be tilted at an angle, providing more resistance, forcing you to burn off more

A TREADMILL IS A GOOD PIECE OF EQUIPMENT TO HAVE IF YOU PLAN TO WORKOUT AT HOME.

SHAPING A TIGHT
& TRIM LOWER BODY

Hot Legs!

calories of fat – which is what you want when shaping a tight and trim lower body.

An exercise that is closely related to walking and also adds a mix of stepping is hiking. Hiking is not always a possibility but it is a great way to work your legs, burn off fat calories, and enjoy the outdoors, all at the same time. One of the nice effects of hiking is that you usually don't realize how much energy you are expending due to the enjoyment of the scenery. Hiking can be a great supplemental exercise if you have the chance.

> ## A MINIMAL NUMBER OF WORKOUTS IS BETTER THAN NO WORKOUTS!

BIKE RIDING

Bike riding is a great way to burn off fat and really gives the legs a good workout. Bike riding can be performed inside on a stationary bike, or outside on a regular bike. Both work the legs well, and use fat for fuel. As noted in the September 1995 issue of *Muscle Media 2000*, fitness star Tatiana Anderson bikes for 45 minutes a day to stay in shape. Miss Galaxy, Ursula Alberto, is noted in the same issue as using a bike in her training. Bike riding on a consistent basis will help you build an incredible lower body.

Cynthia Hill avoids hard surfaces when she runs as a means of injury prevention.

RUNNING

Running is an exercise that will burn off a lot of fat and increase the muscularity of your legs, however, there is a caution. It should not be the main cardio/aerobic exercise in your routine. Running too much, especially on hard surfaces, can lead to leg injuries and set your training back. In spite of this problem, you should not ignore running as it does provide great benefits for your legs and your entire body. The

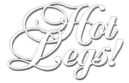

best way to incorporate running into your program is to do it occasionally, perhaps once a week, in addition to your other exercises.

AEROBICS

Specific aerobics, such as "step" aerobics or dance aerobics, incorporate a lot of leg action, and they are a good manner in which to get the combined effects of cardio/aerobic exercise and leg involvement. This form of exercise should be performed continuously for at least 20 minutes to realize a good physical return for your effort.

JUMPING ROPE

A jump-rope workout is great for attaining cardio/aerobic benefits and toning the leg muscles, provided you do not jump on a hard surface, or perform this exercise too often. Jumping rope on a hard surface and jumping too frequently can lead to shin splints and other leg injuries.

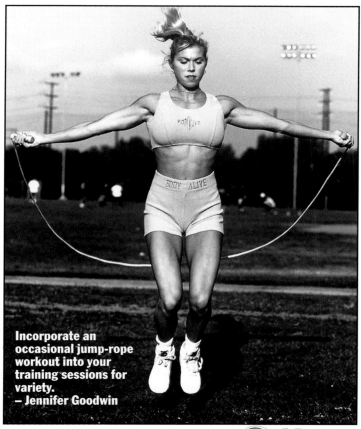

Incorporate an occasional jump-rope workout into your training sessions for variety.
— Jennifer Goodwin

Jumping rope, if you choose to use this form of workout, should be performed on a surface that has some give to it, and not used as the sole exercise in your routine. If you follow these guidelines jumping rope will work well for you.

These are just a few of the many possible cardio/aerobic workouts. The cardio/aerobic workouts that have been mentioned are some of the best, particularly when you consider the involvement of the legs. When choosing an exercise for cardio/aerobic stimulation, pick one of the exercises that have been highlighted. You can use others, but the ones listed work especially well for building the various muscles of your legs.

WEEKLY CARDIO/AEROBIC WORKOUTS

You should consistently get in a few cardio/aerobic workouts every week. A good goal to aim for is 3 to 5 cardio/aerobic workouts of no less than 20 minutes per workout, and preferably 30 to 45 minutes per workout. Not everyone will have the opportunity to get in that many workouts but remember that some workouts are better than no workouts! Some weeks may be better than others for exercising but

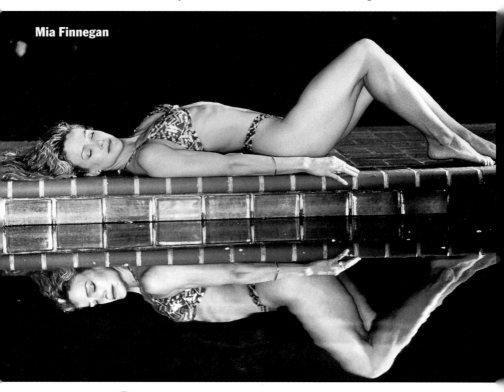

Mia Finnegan

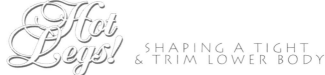

SHAPING A TIGHT
& TRIM LOWER BODY

always attempt to get in some training. Even one cardiovascular workout per week is better than doing nothing. But by all means try to get in more than a couple of cardio/aerobic workouts per week.

VARIETY

You can choose to use just one of these various cardio/aerobic exercises, or you can use a combination of them. You may want to perform only power-walking exercises, or you may want to just use stair-stepping exercises. One idea is to use an anchor exercise, such as stair stepping, which you perform 2 to 3 times a week, and to also use an alternate exercise, such as power walking, jumping rope, aerobics, etc., which you perform 1 to 2 times a week. Or you might try something different each time you work out – rotating through

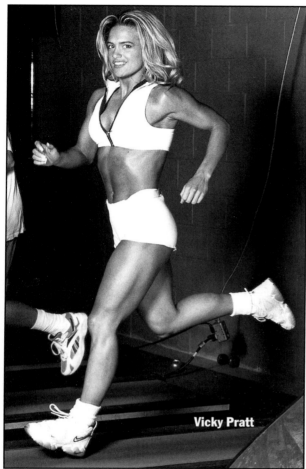

Vicky Pratt

various cardio/aerobic exercises. Variety is the spice of life, and a good way to beat any workout boredom you might encounter in your training program. Exercise choice is a variable that is up to you. The constants in the equation have been noted before – the workouts should last for at least 20 minutes of nonstop action, and should be performed at least 2 or more times per week.

> **VARIETY IS THE SPICE OF LIFE – AND A GOOD WAY TO BEAT WORKOUT BOREDOM!**

Tonya Knight points out additional advice in a *MuscleMag International* article, "Cardio, when done on an empty stomach, is the best way to turn up the heat (for burning fat). This will get your metabolism going and get your body to burn up its fat stores."

SHAPING A TIGHT
& TRIM LOWER BODY

Hot Legs!

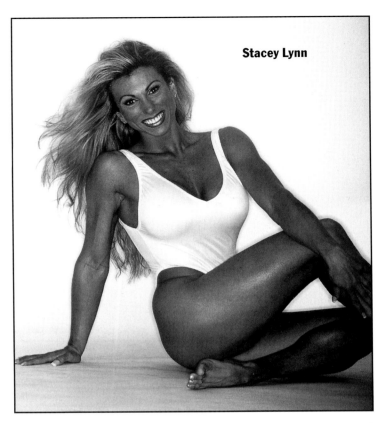

Stacey Lynn

Warm up before each workout, stretching a little and loosening your body up. Get into the workout mentally, and make a commitment to getting all the way through the workout. Have a couple or more glasses of water when you finish to replenish your body.

TOTAL LEG-TRAINING

The cardio/aerobic aspect is an essential element in your *Hot Legs!* program. You can build awesome legs without cardio/aerobic workouts, but the cardio/aerobic workouts add refinement, and make your legs look better than if you just used weight training. Additionally, there are many other benefits realized by cardio/aerobic training, besides accelerating the rate at which you can shape your legs into hot legs! These health benefits of cardio/aerobic training need to be taken into consideration. Neglect of cardio/aerobic exercise can be detrimental to your health, no matter how hot your legs look.

If you want to build the best pair of legs possible, use both weight training and cardio/aerobic exercise. These two elements will really shape your lower body. Part six integrates these two training components.

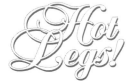

SHAPING A TIGHT & TRIM LOWER BODY

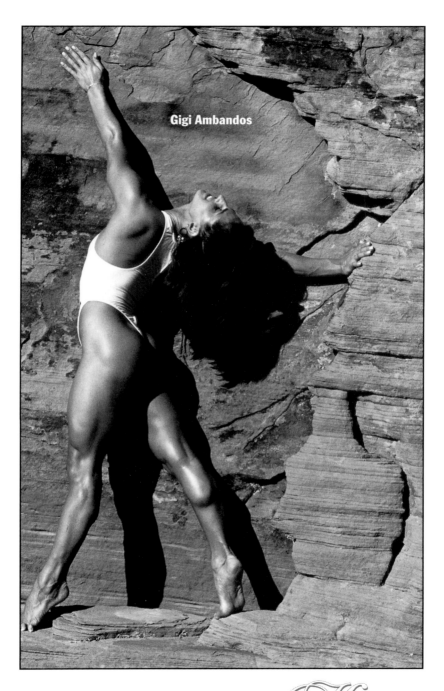

Gigi Ambandos

Part Six
TOTAL LEG-TRAINING

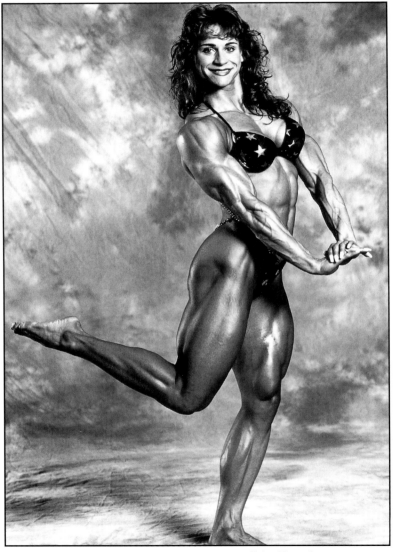

Jitka Harazimova

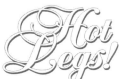

SHAPING A TIGHT
& TRIM LOWER BODY

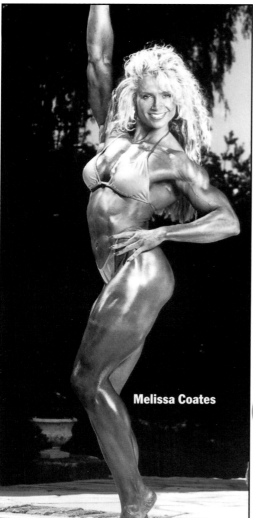

Melissa Coates

The combination of weight training and cardio/aerobic exercise really shapes the legs into fantastic condition. Each of these two elements play a major part in reaching the leg's full potential. By incorporating both elements into a routine you can take control of the condition of your legs and reshape them into the shape you want – tight and trim. The focus of this booklet is on total leg-training – weight training and cardio/aerobic exercises, and how to bring them together to build a great pair of legs.

PRIORITY TRAINING

Not everyone is born with a perfect pair of legs, but there is hope – the shape of the legs can be significantly altered. It is exercise that reshapes the legs, and that is why you have to work on them if you desire change. Since not

> **PRIORITY TRAINING HELPS TO OVERCOME THE WEAK POINTS IN YOUR LEGS.**

everyone is born with perfect legs it pays to find out where your weak points are and make them a priority in your training. Some people have upper thighs that readily respond to training. Others have hamstrings that respond well, while their lower thighs lag. Yet others have calves that really respond to training, but their hamstrings don't. And some need work on each area of their legs. The way to handle any of these problems is priority training – giving priority to the weak points in your legs.

Often the best training is performed at the beginning of your workout, and the best way to prioritize your training is to work your weak areas first. Additional emphasis can be placed on your weak points by performing more work (more sets) than on the other areas of your legs.

SHAPING A TIGHT & TRIM LOWER BODY

Hot Legs!

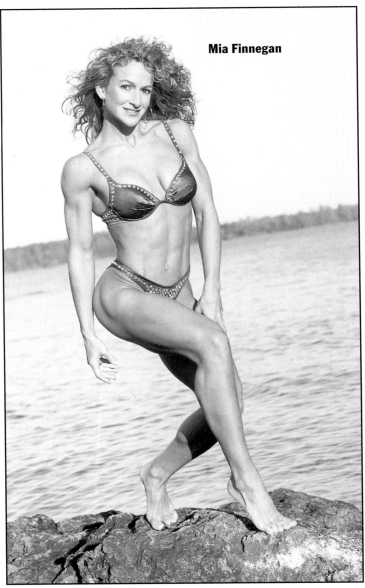

Mia Finnegan

The *Hot Legs!* program provides some general leg-training outlines, and also some priority-training outlines. If you find that some part of your lower body needs additional emphasis, you can choose the priority training that meets your needs. The priority training is broken down into three areas – thigh priority, hamstring priority, and calf priority. The goal is to train your legs to the degree where all three

Hot Legs!

SHAPING A TIGHT
& TRIM LOWER BODY

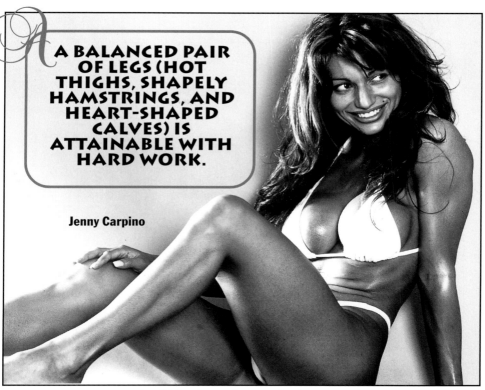

Jenny Carpino

areas – the thighs, hamstrings, and calves – are balanced in their appearance, and where your legs have no weak points. But that is the end goal, and you may have to use priority training to get there. Fitness star Mia Finnegan used priority training to assist in her quest to become the first Fitness Olympia winner. In *Muscle & Fitness* (January 1996) she said, "Recognizing that my quadriceps (thighs) were already big enough, I limited myself to doing only leg extensions to squeeze out the shape and tone I needed." She also used tons of standing and lying leg curls for her hamstrings. Mia was making her hamstrings a priority because her thighs were already good enough. Former multi-Ms. Olympia Lenda Murray noted that she was satisfied with her glutes and hamstrings, but wanted to do plenty of calf work (*Flex*, August 1992). This is another example of a top physique star using priority training. You may also need to work on a particular area of your legs more than another. On the other hand, your entire leg region may need work, or your legs may be fairly well-balanced but need a little more muscle tone. You can use the general training routine if this is the case. Once you have balanced your legs through priority training (if necessary) you can use the general leg-training routines to maintain them in good condition.

GENERAL LEG-TRAINING ROUTINES

WORKOUT 1

Exercise	Sets	Reps
Squats	2	10
Stiff-leg Deadlifts	2	10
Standing Calf Raises	2	10

WORKOUT 2

Exercise	Sets	Reps
Hack Squats	3	8
Leg Curls	2	12
Seated Calf Raises	3	10

WORKOUT 3

Exercise	Sets	Reps
Leg Extensions	1	10
Sissy Squats	2	10
Stiff-leg Deadlifts	2	12
Standing Dumbell Calf Raises	2	15

WORKOUT 4

Exercise	Sets	Reps
Squats	1	12
Lunges	2	12
Cable Leg Curls	2	10
Seated Calf Raises	3	10

WORKOUT 5

Exercise	Sets	Reps
Roman-chair Squats	2	10
Hack Squats	1	12
Stiff-leg Deadlifts	2	10
Standing Calf Raises	2	15

WORKOUT 6

Exercise	Sets	Reps
Leg Extensions	3	15
Standing Leg Curls	2	15
Seated Calf Raises	3	12

Always warm up without weights before working out, going through the same motions of the exercise you will be performing.

The various workouts in the general workout section are interchangeable and provide a general guideline from which to get you started. Feel free to change the

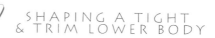

SHAPING A TIGHT
& TRIM LOWER BODY

various exercises around, substituting what works for you for what doesn't. The same holds true for the repetition and set range. Generally work within a 8- to 15-rep range per exercise for 2 to 3 sets.

These workouts should be performed 1 to 2 times a week, with at least 2 days of rest between each leg workout. It is important to give your legs a day or more off from weight training so they can fully recover.

Cardio/aerobic training is to be integrated into these weight-training programs. Perform 2 to 5 cardio/aerobic workouts per week along with these weight-training exercises. When you start training you will probably get into the best workout groove by easing into the routine. Start with one weight-training workout for the legs, and a couple of cardio/aerobic workouts. You might want to do a cardio/aerobic workout on Monday (stair stepping, power walking, etc.), a weight training workout on Wednesday, and another cardio/aerobic workout on Friday. As your body becomes accustomed to the work-

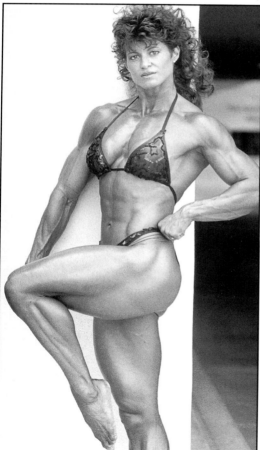

load gradually add a little more cardio/aerobic work to your weekly routine. Aim for at least 3 cardio/aerobic workouts per week, and get in more if you can. Your body will tell you when you have reached your limit. When you get to this point (too many workouts) you should reduce your weekly routine by one cardio/aerobic workout. Keep your weight training for your legs at a steady 1 to 2 workouts per week, but do not go beyond this frequency level! It is too easy to overtrain when it comes to weight training. You can handle (and your body needs) more cardio/aerobic work. You can perform cardio/aerobic work on the same day as you perform weight training. Some people like to perform a weight-training workout for their legs, and then get on a treadmill or stair stepper after the workout. Others take a long walk. The sequence of your cardio/aerobic workouts is up to you, depending on your individual needs.

Joanne McCartney

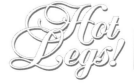

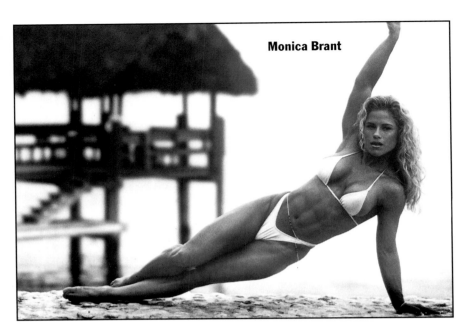

Monica Brant

PRIORITY WORKOUTS

CALF PRIORITY

WORKOUT 1

Exercises	Sets	Reps
Seated Calf Raises	3	12
Standing Calf Raises	2	10
Squats	1	15
Leg Curls	2	10

WORKOUT 2

Exercises	Sets	Reps
Dumbell Standing Calf Raises	3	10
Seated Calf Raises	2	15
Hack Squats	1	12
Stiff-leg Deadlifts	1	10

WORKOUT 3

Exercises	Sets	Reps
Standing Calf Raises	4	12
One-leg Calf Raises, no weight	2	20-25
Leg Extensions	1	15
Standing Leg Curls	1	12

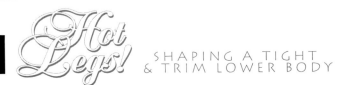

SHAPING A TIGHT
& TRIM LOWER BODY

These workouts will really help if you need to pay particular attention to your calves. The amount of work for the other muscle groups is reduced while the work for the calves is increased. The workout routines are not "hard and fast" – you can make some changes to meet your needs, but perform at least twice as many sets for the calves as you do for the other exercises, and perform the calf exercises first in the workout sequence. Also place the stretching, flexing and tightening emphasis (between sets) on the calves.

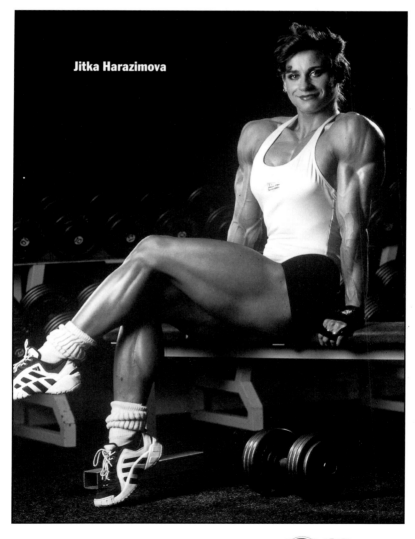

Jitka Harazimova

HAMSTRING PRIORITY

WORKOUT 1

Exercises	Sets	Reps
Leg Curls	2	12
Stiff-leg Deadlifts	3	10
Leg Extensions	1	15
Seated Calf Raises	2	10

WORKOUT 2

Exercises	Sets	Reps
Stiff-leg Deadlifts	4	12
Lunges	1	15
Standing Calf Raises	1	12

WORKOUT 3

Exercises	Sets	Reps
Standing Leg Curls	2	12
Stiff-leg Deadlifts	1	12
Cable Leg Curls	2	10
Hack Squats	1	8
One-Leg Dumbell Calf Raises	2	12

These workouts place primary emphasis on the hamstrings. Tighten the hamstring muscles repeatedly between sets. As mentioned you can rotate various exercises around and experiment with the repetition and set arrangement, but always keep the majority of sets centered around hamstring work when you are focusing on hamstring priority training.

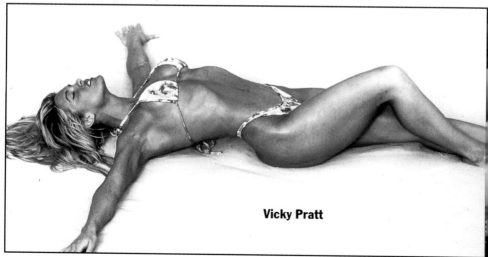

Vicky Pratt

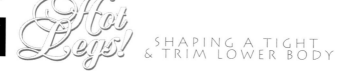

SHAPING A TIGHT
& TRIM LOWER BODY

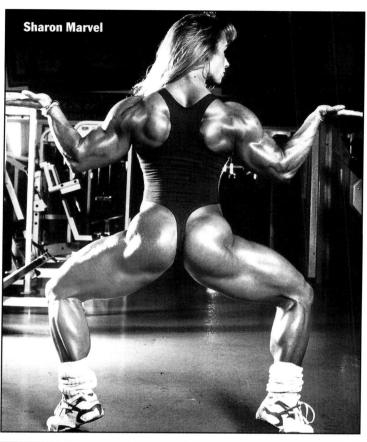

Sharon Marvel

THIGH PRIORITY
WORKOUT 1

Exercises	Sets	Reps
Squats	3	10
Leg Extensions	2	15
Leg Curls	1	15
Seated Calf Raises	1	15

WORKOUT 2

Exercises	Sets	Reps
Sissy Squats	3	10
Hack Squats	2	10
Stiff-leg Deadlifts	1	12
Standing Calf Raises	2	12

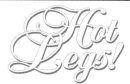

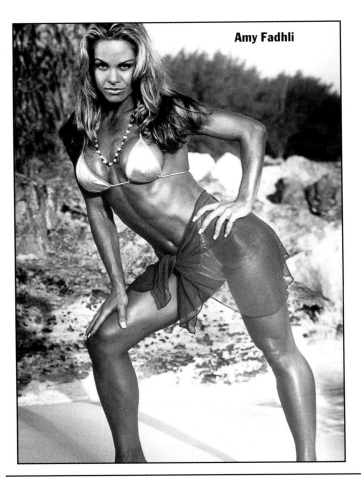

Amy Fadhli

WORKOUT 3

Exercises	Sets	Reps
Squats	2	20
Roman-chair Squats	2	10
Cable Leg Curls	1	12
Seated Calf Raises	1	20

WORKOUT 4

Exercises	Sets	Reps
Hack Squats	2	12
Lunges	1	10
Sissy Squats	2	15
Stiff-leg Deadlifts	1	15
Standing Calf Raises	2	12

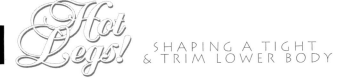

When using priority training for the thighs make the thigh exercises the central focus of your workout, and make use of more sets. Stretch the thighs out well before and after the workout, and contract the muscles tightly between sets.

Priority training enables you to direct the effort of your workout right where you want it. Use the workouts as guidelines for improving your legs. Remember, these are only guidelines, and if you feel you need more or less work in some area of your leg development (more or less exercises, sets, repetitions, etc.), then follow what your body is telling you. Check out your legs in the mirror and see what areas need improvement. Put the emphasis of your leg-training on those area(s). Note which part of your legs are better, and don't need as much attention. As with the general leg-training workouts,

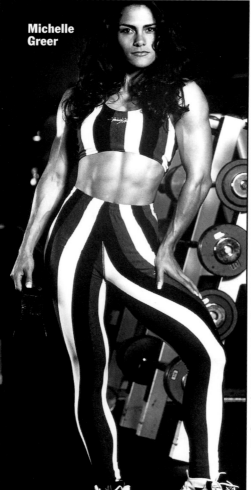

Michelle Greer

also include cardio/aerobic work with the priority-training workout. Use the same guidelines as with the general leg-training workouts – at least a couple of cardio/ aerobic workouts (lasting more than 20 minutes) per week, and preferably more than that. Also remember to give your leg muscles a couple of days of rest before working them with weights again.

LEG-GROUP ROTATION

There is no law that says you have to work all of the leg muscles together. Most people just find this approach to be very practical and quick. As noted in *MuscleMag International*, Dinah Anderson uses one day to focus on training her legs. So does Marjo Selin. Kathy Unger performs her thigh workouts one day, and her hamstrings and calves on a different day (*Natural Bodybuilding*, May 1996).

You can use whatever approach you want to. You can work each leg muscle on a different day if you choose (for example – thighs on Monday, hamstrings on Wednesday, and calves on Friday). This approach will allow you to have the energy to perform a couple of extra sets for each bodypart. You can also use a rotation with priority training. For instance, if you were focusing on calves as your priority, you might work calves on Monday, and thighs and hamstrings on Wednesday. This would allow you to really blast the calves in one workout. You have all kinds of options for working your legs. Just remember that when it comes to weight training, it is crucial to give each individual muscle group a couple of days off before working it again.

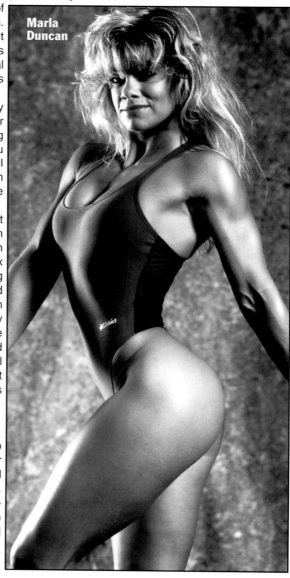

Marla Duncan

Leg-training isn't easy – it will take an iron will on your part to tame your legs, making them conform to the shape you want them to be. But they will yield if you are consistent with your workouts and follow the guidelines in *Hot Legs!*

You can compliment your leg-training program with a nutritious diet. An increase in quality protein and complex carbohydrates and fibers along with a decrease in fat and sugar will greatly aid you in your quest for fit and healthy legs. An increase in your intake of water, along with a good one-a-day vitamin and mineral supplement will also assist your body in transforming its appearance.

HOT LEGS!

Use the *Hot Legs!* program to guide you in reshaping your legs, making them tighter and trimmer than they are now. Gradually work into the program. Experiment with the various training routines until

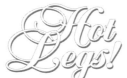

SHAPING A TIGHT & TRIM LOWER BODY

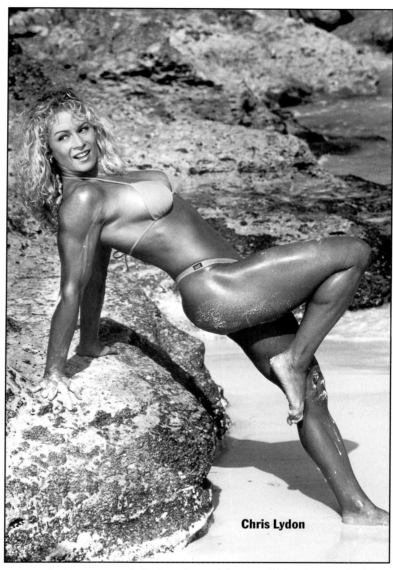

Chris Lydon

you find an approach that works well for you. Listen to your body's response and react to it. Fitness star Nancy Georges uses this approach – she uses different exercises, finding out which ones feel like they are working and which ones don't (*Ironman*, September 1994). Be willing to change things now. If you pay close attention to the information and guidelines presented in this booklet you can shape a tight and trim lower body.

The hot legs you desire don't have to be a dream – they can be a reality!

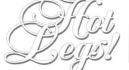

SHAPING A TIGHT
& TRIM LOWER BODY

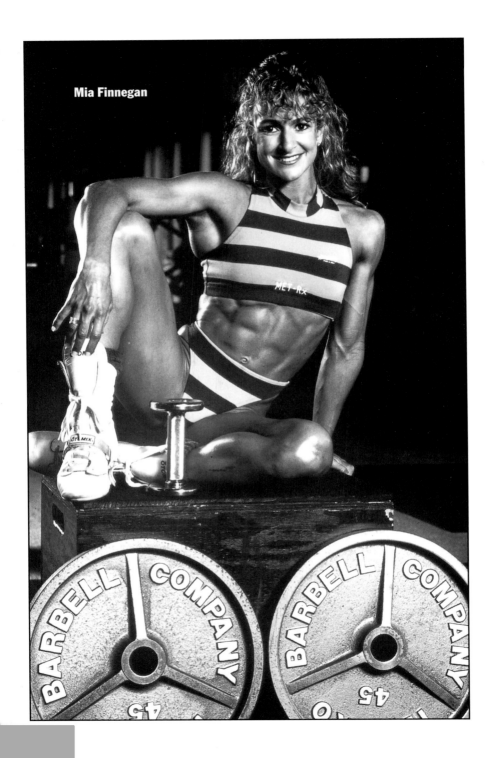

Mia Finnegan

Contributing Photographers

Jim Amentler, Alex Ardenti,
Reg Bradford, Skip Faulkner,
Irvin Gelb, Richard Finnegan,
Robert Kennedy, Marconi,
Jason Mathas, John Running